TETRAPLEGIA

EXPLORING THE WORLD OF CURING

TETRAPLEGIA

DR. CYRIL LAKES

Table of Contents

CHAPTER ONE

INTRODUCTION

A spinal cord injury can be caused by any lesion to the spinal cord or the nerves at the end of the spinal canal. These injuries often leave long-term changes in strength, sensation, and other body functions below the site of the injury.

It could seem like everything in your life will change if you recently had a spinal cord injury.

Many scientists believe that spinal cord injuries will be able to be repaired in the future because to scientific developments. Research is still being done on a global scale. Thanks to therapy and rehabilitation, many people with spinal cord injuries are able to lead independent, productive lives in the interim.

Signs and symptoms

How well you are able to control your limbs after a spinal cord injury depends on the location and severity of the injury along your spinal cord.

The lowest part of your spinal cord that remains functional after an injury is known as the neurological level of impairment. The term "the completeness" refers to the extent of damage, which can be divided into two categories:

completed. If almost all motor function (control) and sensory perception (sensation) are lost below the spinal cord lesion, your injury is deemed complete.

Not quite finished. If you still have some motor or sensory function below the injured area, your injury is classified as partial. There are various degrees of partial damage.

Moreover, paralysis brought on by injury to the spinal cord may be referred to as:

Tetraplegia. This disorder, which is also known as quadriplegia, denotes that your arms, hands, trunk, legs, and pelvic organs have all been impacted by spinal cord damage.

Immobility. This paralysis affects all or part of the trunk, pelvic organs, and legs.

Your healthcare team will perform a series of tests to determine the degree and neurological condition of your injury.

One or more of the following signs and symptoms could be the result of any kind of spinal cord injury:

Reduction in movement

loss of sensibility, including touch, humidity, and temperature

loss of bowel or bladder control

increased contractions or reflex actions

changes to sexual sensitivity, fertility, and sexual function a terrible stinging sensation or pain brought on by damage to the nerve fibers in your spinal cord

difficulties breathing, coughing, or clearing your lungs of mucus

Emergency warning signs and symptoms

Emergency signs and symptoms of a spinal cord injury after an accident may include:

Extreme pressure in your neck, back, or head, or soreness in your back

Any part of your body that seems weak, paralyzed, or uncoordinated

You can feel numbness, tingling, or loss of feeling in your hands, fingers, feet, or toes.

A decline in bladder or bowel control

Difficulty walking and keeping your balance

Breathing issues after a trauma

A crooked or twisted back or neck

When to see a doctor

To rule out potential spinal injuries, anyone with serious head or neck trauma should see a doctor very away. In actuality, it is safest to assume that trauma patients have spinal injury unless the opposite is proven because:

Not every serious spinal injury manifests itself right away. If it is ignored, more severe damage might occur.

Numbness or paralysis may happen suddenly or gradually when there is hemorrhage or edema in or around the spinal cord.

The amount of time that passes between an injury and the onset of therapy can have a substantial impact on both the length of recovery and the severity of consequences.

If you suspect a person may have had a back or neck injury:

Maintain the injured person's immobility to avoid permanent paralysis and other potentially fatal consequences.

Press the emergency medical assistance number in your region or 911.

Keep the person still.

To prevent the head and neck from moving until emergency help arrives, either hold them in place or cover them with large towels.

Assist the patient with basic first aid, such as stopping any bleeding and providing comfort, without moving their head or neck.

Motives

Spinal cord injuries can be caused by injury to the spinal cord itself or to the vertebrae, ligaments, or disks that make up the spinal column.

Traumatic spinal cord injury can occur from a sudden, strong blow to the spine that fractures, dislocates, crushes, or compresses one or more vertebrae. It might also be the result of a spinal cord piercing and cutting caused by a knife or bullet trauma.

Extra damage usually appears over a few days or weeks due to edema, inflammation, fluid accumulation, and bleeding in and around the spinal cord.

Nontraumatic spinal cord injuries can be caused by degenerative disk degeneration in the spine, arthritis, cancer, infections, and inflammation.

Your brain and central nervous system

The central nervous system is made up of the brain and spinal cord. The spinal cord, which extends downward from the base of your brain, is made up of nerve cells and soft tissue. These cells are arranged into tracts that link to different parts of your body. Vertebrae ring the spinal cord.

The region right above your waist where the lower end of your spinal cord ends is called the conus medullaris. Below this region lies a group of nerve roots called the cauda equina.

There are tracts in your spinal cord that carry messages from your brain to the different areas of your body. The motor tracts receive signals from the brain that control how muscles move. The brain receives information from many body areas via sensory pathways regarding pressure, temperature, discomfort, and limb posture.

Damage to the nerve fibers passing through the injured area, regardless of their source, affects them and can either totally or partially impair the corresponding muscles and nerves below the site of the injury.

A lumbar or thoracic spine injury can affect the legs, torso, bowel and bladder control, and sexual function. Your arms' range of motion is also impacted by a cervical (neck) injury, which may even make breathing difficult.

Most common causes of spinal cord injury

The most common causes of spinal cord injuries in the United States are:

auto mishaps. Auto and motorcycle accidents are the primary cause of spinal cord injury, accounting for around 35 percent of new cases each year.

crumbles. Falls are the leading cause of spinal cord injury in adults over 65. Overall, falls are the cause of more than 25% of spinal cord injuries.

violent deeds. Roughly 15% of spinal cord injuries are caused by violent situations, which often involve gunshot and knife wounds, according to the National Spinal Cord Injury Statistical Center.

injuries incurred when doing sports or relaxing. Roughly 9% of spinal cord injuries are related to sports, such as impact sports and shallow water diving.

alcohol. Alcohol use is the cause of about one in four spinal cord injury.

ailments. Rheumatoid arthritis, osteoporosis, malignancy, and spinal cord inflammation can potentially cause spinal cord damage.

Hazardous components

While spinal cord injuries are usually the result of accidents and can happen to anybody, several factors can increase your risk of suffering one, including:

being a male. A greater number of spinal cord injuries occur in men. In fact, women account for just about 20% of traumatic spinal cord injuries in the United States.

Being between the ages of 16 and 30. A person between the ages of 16 and 30 is more prone to suffer a catastrophic spinal cord injury.

Being older than sixty-five. Falls account for the majority of injuries sustained by the elderly.

Engaging in risky pursuits. Engaging in sports or diving into extremely shallow water without wearing the proper safety gear or taking the essential precautions can cause spinal cord injury. Motor vehicle accidents are the primary cause of spinal cord injury in individuals under 65.

suffering from a disease of the bones or joints. A fairly minor injury may cause spinal cord damage if you have osteoporosis, arthritis, or any other ailment that affects your bones or joints.

VOUCHERS

At first, the changes in how your body functions could be too much to handle. That being said, your rehabilitation team will help you make the preparations you need to deal with the changes brought about by the spinal cord injury. Frequently affected regions consist of:

bladder control. Your bladder will continue to hold on to pee from your kidneys. But your brain may not be able to control your bladder as well if injury occurs to the spinal cord, which serves as the communication pathway.

The decreased control over the bladder increases the risk of urinary tract infections. They can lead to kidney infections as well as kidney or bladder stones.

During your rehabilitation, you will learn new techniques to assist you in passing urine.

intestinal control. Even if you regularly have altered control over your bowel motions, your stomach and intestines continue to function essentially the same.

CHAPTER TWO

You'll learn how to optimize your bowel movements and maintain a high-fiber diet to help keep your intestines in check during your recovery.

Skin sensation. It's possible that some or all of your skin's sensations have disappeared beneath the damage to your nervous system. Your skin cannot thus communicate with your brain when it is injured by something, such as constant pressure, heat, or cold.

This may make you more susceptible to pressure sores, but you can reduce your risk by changing positions frequently and getting aid if needed. You will learn how to properly care for your skin during rehabilitation, which may help you avoid these problems.

Control of the flow. Spinal cord injuries can cause a variety of circulatory problems, such as low blood pressure upon standing up and edema in your extremities. These changes to circulation may also increase the risk of deep vein thrombosis and pulmonary emboli, two types of blood clots.

Another problem with circulation control is autonomic hyperreflexia, which can result in a potentially lethal rise in blood pressure. Your rehabilitation team will teach you coping skills if these problems affect you.

breathing apparatus. Breathing and coughing may become more difficult if your injuries affect the muscles in your chest and abdomen. Among these are the diaphragm and the muscles in your abdomen and chest wall.

The degree of your neurological damage will determine the kind of respiratory problems you may encounter. An damage to the thoracic and cervical spinal cords may increase your risk of developing lung problems such as pneumonia. Counseling and medication are effective treatments for these problems.

muscular tone. Some people with spinal cord injuries experience two sorts of problems with muscle tone: flaccidity, which is characterized by soft, limp muscles devoid of muscular tone, and spasticity, which is an uncontrolled tightening or twitching of the muscles.

wellness and overall health. Weight loss and muscular atrophy are common after a spinal cord injury. Reduced mobility leads to a more sedentary lifestyle, which raises your risk of obesity, diabetes, and cardiovascular disease.

You can follow a dietician's recommended diet to stay at a healthy weight. You can get help from physical and occupational therapists in developing an exercise and fitness program.

sexual health. Sexual function, fertility, and sexuality may be affected by spinal cord injury. Men may report differences in erection and ejaculation, while women may notice changes in lubrication.

Specialists in spinal cord injury in medicine, urology, and reproductive health can offer options for sexual functioning and fertility.

agony. Some people have joint or muscular pain as a result of overusing particular muscle groups. Nerve pain, also known as neuropathic or central pain, can arise following a spinal cord injury, especially in individuals with incomplete injuries.

Depression. Living with pain and adjusting to all the changes brought about by a spinal cord injury can cause depression in some people.

Treatment options for depression resulting from a spinal cord injury include counseling and medication.

Getting Ready for the Meeting

Emergency spinal cord injuries can prevent the patient from participating in their own care at first.

Multiple specialists will be needed to stabilize the situation, including a physician with experience in nerve system problems (neurologist) and a surgeon with experience in spinal cord injuries and other nervous system issues (neurosurgeon).

The rehabilitation program's multidisciplinary team will be led by a physician with specialized training in spinal cord injury.

If you think you may have a spinal cord injury, or if you know someone who has and can't provide the information needed, here are some things you may do to help with care.

What you're able to accomplish

Even if the events don't seem related, be prepared to provide facts about the occurrence that resulted in the injury.

Ask a friend or family member to accompany you when you speak with the doctors, if at all possible. Sometimes it could be difficult to remember everything that was said. A friend or relative might be able to recollect the details and help you communicate them to the injured individual at the appropriate time.

Make a list of questions for the doctors.

The following are some basic questions to ask the physician regarding a spinal cord injury:

What is the prognosis?

What are the current plans in place? What will eventually happen? Which treatment option would you recommend?

What kinds of side effects are usual when receiving treatment?

Would having surgery be advantageous?

What kind of treatment might be helpful?

Are there any alternatives to the primary tactic you suggest?

Which research projects are being undertaken to address this issue?

Are there any printed items you have, like brochures? Are there any websites you would recommend?

Ask away with any other queries you may have.

What to expect from the doctor

Your physician will probably ask you about the following:

What particular incidents led to your injury?

What time did it occur?

What is your source of income?

With whom do you live?

Does anyone in your family have a history of blood clots?

Do you have any other ailments at the moment?

Examinations and diagnosis

An ER doctor may be able to rule out a spinal cord damage with a thorough examination, mobility and sensory function tests, and questions about the trauma.

However, if the injured party complains of neck pain, is not fully awake, or shows obvious signs of neurological damage or weakening, then urgent diagnostic testing might be necessary.

These tests might include the following:

CT scan stands for computed tomography. Sometimes a CT scan might reveal abnormalities more clearly than an X-ray. In this scan, a series of cross-sectional images that can detect disk, bone, and other problems are produced by computers.

radiography. Medical practitioners typically seek these tests when they suspect a patient has had trauma and may have suffered a spinal cord damage. X-rays can detect issues in the vertebral column, degenerative changes in the spine, and cancers.

Magnetic resonance imaging is referred to as MRI. MRI uses a strong magnetic field and radio waves to produce computer-generated images. This test is very useful for examining the spinal cord in order to find any masses, such as blood clots or herniated disks, that may be compressing the spinal cord.

A few days following the incident, maybe after some of the swelling has subsided, your doctor will do a neurological exam to determine the amount and kind of your injury. This tests your sensitivity to light touch and a pinprick as well as your muscle strength.

CHAPTER THREE

Drugs and supplements

Regretfully, spinal cord injuries are irreversible. But researchers are always coming up with new treatments, such prosthetic limbs and medications, that could promote nerve cell regeneration or improve the functionality of the nerves that survive spinal cord injury.

While this is happening, the aim of treating spinal cord injuries is to prevent further harm and allow patients who have had one to resume active, rewarding lives.

The impact of any head or neck injuries must be minimized, and this requires quick medical attention. For this reason, spinal cord injury therapy often begins at the scene of the crash.

Emergency personnel will typically use a stiff neck collar and rigid carrying board to immobilize your spine as quickly and gently as possible while transferring you to the hospital.

The first (acute) stages of treatment

Doctors in the ER give priority to:

Holding on to your breath

Preventing shock

Maintaining immobility of the neck to prevent further spinal cord damage

avoiding possible adverse effects include heartburn or breathing difficulties, urine or feces retention, and the formation of deep vein blood clots in the limbs

You may be put under anesthesia during diagnostic tests for a spinal cord injury in order to keep you from moving and injuring yourself more.

If you do sustain a spinal cord injury, you will usually be admitted to the intensive care unit for treatment. You might even be paired with a team at a regional spine injury center that includes orthopedic surgeons, neurosurgeons, spinal cord injury specialists, psychologists, nurses, therapists, and social workers.

medicines. One treatment option for acute spinal cord injury is intravenous (IV) methylprednisolone (A-Methapred, Solu-Medrol). In certain cases, people who get methylprednisolone within eight hours of the injury show a moderate improvement.

It appears to work by reducing damage to nerve cells and inflammation around the site of injury. On the other hand, it is not a spinal cord injury treatment.

motionlessness. To properly align your spine, stabilize it, or do both, you might need traction. A stiff neck collar could be helpful in some circumstances. A particular bed can also render your body immobile.

surgery. Surgery is often necessary to remove foreign objects, fractured vertebrae, herniated disks, and broken bone pieces that appear to be crushing the spine. Surgery may also be necessary to stabilize the spine and prevent discomfort or deformity in the future.

experimental techniques. Scientists are trying to come up with ways to control inflammation, promote neuron regeneration, and stop cell death. Find out whether these treatments are available from your doctor.

Constant attention

Once the initial injury or illness has stabilized, doctors concentrate on preventing potential secondary complications such as muscle contractures, deconditioning, pressure ulcers, bowel and bladder issues, lung infections, and blood clots.

Your condition and the medical issues you are facing will dictate how long you stay in the hospital. When you recover enough to participate in therapies and treatments, you could go to a rehabilitation facility.

Healing

Early on in your recovery, you will begin working with members of the rehabilitation team. On your team may be occupational therapists, physical therapists, social workers, nutritionists, rehabilitation psychologists, rehabilitation nurses, and physiatrists, doctors who specialize in physical medicine or spinal cord injuries.

Early on in the healing process, therapists usually focus on developing adaptive methods for everyday chores, restoring fine motor abilities, and maintaining and improving previous muscle function.

You will get advice on getting your life back on track and enhancing your quality of life, as well as knowledge on the potential complications of a spinal cord injury.

You will learn a lot of new skills and utilize equipment and technology to help you live as independently as possible. Resuming your favorite activities, returning to social and physical activities, and returning to work or school will all be encouraged.

Medications

Medication can help manage certain adverse effects that may arise from a spinal cord injury. These include medications that improve bowel, bladder, and sexual function in addition to those that lessen pain and muscular stiffness.

Innovative technologies

Innovative medical technologies can help people with spinal cord injuries become more mobile and independent. Some devices may also revert to factory settings. Among them are:

modern wheelchairs. With the advent of lighter, more advanced wheelchairs, people with spinal cord injuries are becoming more mobile and comfortable. It's possible that some people need an electric wheelchair. Some wheelchairs can even climb stairs, navigate uneven surfaces, and lift a seated user to eye level so they can independently access high regions.

modifications for computers. For someone with limited hand function, computers can be immensely beneficial tools, even though they can be challenging to use. Key guards and voice recognition are two instances of basic to sophisticated computer modifications.

everyday use of electronic aid. Almost every electrically powered device can be operated by an electronic assistance to daily living (EADL). Devices can be turned on and off via switches, computer-based remotes, and voice-activated remotes.

devices that stimulate electricity. These cutting-edge devices produce motions by electrical stimulation. Known as functional electrical stimulation (FES) systems, these gadgets allow people with spinal cord injuries to reach, grip, stand, and walk by using electrical stimulators to control the muscles in their arms and legs.

instructions for robotic walking. This state-of-the-art device is used to relearn walking abilities following spinal cord injuries.

Diagnosis and recovery

Your doctor may not give you a prognosis straight away. If healing occurs, it often starts one to six months after the injury. Nonetheless, some people do continue to experience modest advantages for a year or more.

CHAPTER FOUR

Homeopathic medicine and lifestyle

By following this advice, you may reduce the likelihood of experiencing a spinal cord injury:

Be careful when driving. Car crashes are among the most common causes of spinal cord injuries. Always wear a seat belt when driving or riding in a car.

Make sure your children are wearing seat belts or using a child safety seat appropriate for their weight and age. To prevent airbag injuries, children under the age of twelve should never ride in the backseat.

Verify the water's depth before diving. Avoid diving into pools that aren't deeper than nine feet, or around three meters, as well as aboveground pools and any body of water whose depth you are unsure of, to be sure you don't end yourself in shallow water.

Prevent falling. Use a step stool with a grab bar if you need to reach high objects. On every staircase, install rails. Put non-slip mats on tile floors and in the bathtub and shower. To prevent little children from accessing the stairs, think about installing window guards and safety gates.

Sports participation should be done with discretion. Always wear the recommended safety equipment. Avoid using your head to lead in sports. For example, you shouldn't slide headfirst in baseball and you shouldn't tackle with your helmet on top in football. Use a spotter when learning new gymnastics moves.

Steer clear of drinking and driving. Never drive while intoxicated or under the influence of drugs. Never take a trip with an intoxicated driver.

Making modifications and providing assistance

A crippling mishap can be a life-changing event. It takes some getting used to having a disability; it might be frightening and confusing to suddenly have one. You could be worried about how your spinal cord injury will affect your relationships with others, your daily life, your career, and your general level of happiness.

Even though recovering from such an event takes time, many people with disabilities go on to lead fulfilling lives. Keeping your motivation high and getting the help you need are essential.

Sadness

If you were recently hurt, you and your family will undoubtedly experience a period of mourning. Although each person's grieving process is different, it's common to experience phases like denial or incredulity, grief, rage, bargaining, and acceptance.

A natural and healthy part of the healing process is grieving. It's acceptable and essential to feel sorrow for the person you used to be. But you also have to figure out how to move forward with your life and establish new plans.

You probably worry about how your injuries may affect your lifestyle, finances, and relationships. Grief and emotional distress are common and acceptable.

But if your grief and depression are getting in the way of your therapy, isolating you from people, or pushing you to abuse alcohol or other drugs, you may want to consider seeing a social worker, psychologist, or psychiatrist. An alternative would be to join a support group specifically for people with spinal cord injuries.

Speaking with others going through similar experiences can be comforting, and group members may have insightful advice on how to rearrange specific areas of your home or office to better meet your needs at the moment. Ask your doctor or a rehabilitation specialist about community support groups.

Taking the lead

One of the best ways to regain control over your life is to learn as much as you can about your injury and your options for leading a more independent life. These days, a wide range of auto accessories and modifications are available.

Similar products are used for home remodeling. Grab bars, wide doors, easy-to-turn doorknobs, customized sinks, and ramps all help you live a more independent life.

The costs of treating a spinal cord injury may be so high that you may want to check to see whether you are eligible for other services or financial aid from the federal, state, or nonprofit sectors. Your rehabilitation team can help you find resources in your area.

Talking about your disability

Your friends and family may respond to your disability in different ways. Some people may experience discomfort and doubt about the appropriateness of what they're saying or doing.

Being willing to teach people and having as much knowledge as possible about your spinal cord injury are beneficial. Children are naturally curious, so if you answer their questions in a clear and understandable way, they could soon adjust. Adults might also benefit from knowing the truth.

Explain the effects of your injury and the methods in which your family can help. Furthermore, if friends and family are helping too much, don't be hesitant to confront them. Although it may not seem comfortable at first, talking to family and friends about your injuries can frequently make things feel better.

Discussing intimacy, sexuality, and having sex

Your spinal cord damage may affect how your body responds to sexual cues. However, you are a sexual being with sexually charged desires. A fulfilling emotional and physical relationship is achievable, but it requires persistence, open communication, and a willingness to try new things.

With the help of a certified counselor, you and your partner may express your desires and emotions more effectively. Your doctor can provide you with the required medical information regarding sexual health. You can have a happy, fulfilled future with lots of sex and connection.

Thinking forward

Naturally, a spinal cord injury has an immediate impact on your life as well as the lives of those closest to you. As soon as you learn you have a diagnosis, you may start mentally cataloging all the things you can no longer do. But when you learn more about your condition and your alternatives for therapy, you might be surprised at what you can do.

Basketball and track meet competitions are now possible for people with spinal cord injuries because to contemporary therapy, tools, and technologies. They paint and take photos. They get married, have children and raise them, and have rewarding careers.

For those suffering from spinal cord injuries, new advancements in stem cell and nerve cell therapy provide hope for a more complete recovery. Concurrent research is being done on new medications for people with chronic spinal cord injuries.

Although no one can tell when new treatments may become available, you may be optimistic about the future of spinal cord research and live life to the fullest right now.

THE END